TIPS AND TRICKS FOR
GOOD PARENTING

How to be a Confident Respectful Modern Parent

Marianne Kind

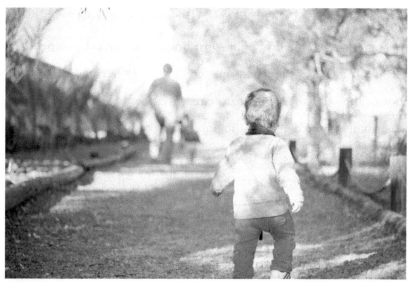

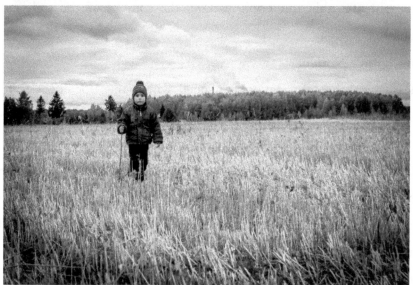

Table of Contents

Chapter 1. Roles of Parents..6

Chapter 2. Positive Parenting Principles 14

Chapter 3. Parenting a Strong-Willed Child 19

Chapter 4. Managing Anger in Children 26

Chapter 5. No More Yelling (How to Teach Without Yelling) 40

Chapter 6. Calm and Confident Leader....................................46

Chapter 7. Common Parenting Mistakes When Training Toddlers.....60

Chapter 8. Children Discipline - Parenting Tips 64

Chapter 9. Parenting Tips for Teaching a Toddler...................70

Chapter 10. Consequences from Improper Training of your Toddlers
....80

Chapter 11. Montesssori Method Managing Choice and Freedom 86

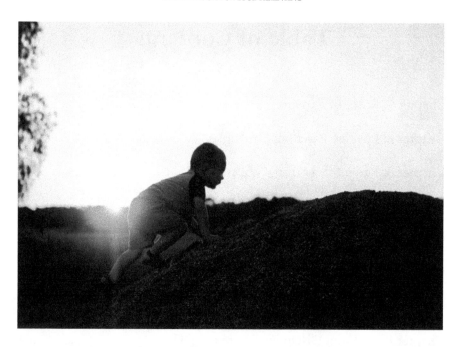

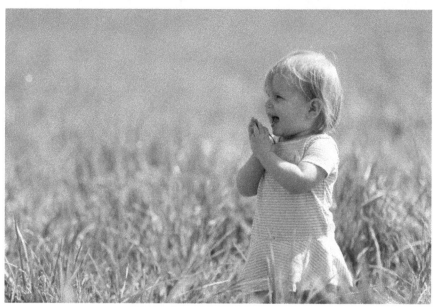

Chapter 1.

Roles of Parents

The most potent desire or drive in man is often his physiological need to fulfill the act of procreation.

We often assume that parenting should come automatically and that we will be better parents than the parents who raised us. Relationships are like rose gardens when well-kept. They are beautiful. But if we leave our relationships un-kept, we will end up with dysfunctional relationships that bring us nothing but stress.

Roles that a Parent Must Focus On

There are six leading roles that a parent must focus on: Love, Guidance, Provision, Security, Friendship, and Development.

Each child is different, and some of them need more attention than others, especially strong-willed children, but we must fulfill our role as parents regardless of the difficulty. One thing all parents must learn is that having children is undoubtedly a life-changing event.

No matter how many children, each child is different and unique with a different set of challenges.

Love

Some parents believe that loving a child will come easy, and for the most part, it does. However, there are moments when love becomes strained, and tempers flare. Maybe the child is not on your schedule and not allowing you to sleep (which happens the first few months of life).

Strong-willed children may often test the boundaries of love. They may often leave you exhausted and even depressed with their antics.

When you become challenged in raising a strong-willed child, try and get help. Even when you are stressed-out from parenting, you still have a responsibility to love the child. If you start to feel the strain, seek help, and try to break it.

But when we talk about love in relationships, we are not just talking exclusively about some sense of mutual endearment or fondness.

Parenting a strong-willed child will require what is referred to as "tough love." As children learn about the world, they live in, and they will often do make choices they shouldn't. As parents, if we love our children, then we must encourage them to do what's right. Sometimes we have a misplaced sense of what love is in parenting, and we focus too much on endearment in times when we are required to show tough love.

When we focus on being liked or loved by our children rather than on encouraging them to do what's right for their good, then it's not them that we love but ourselves.

You must ask yourself, are you sacrificing their long-term fulfillment and happiness in life for your short-term sense of peace and endearment.

When your child takes a jar of jam from the supermarket aisle and smashes it on the floor because you refused to buy a toy for them, what do you do?

However, you choose to correct the behavior is down to you, but you must correct this behavior. Suppose we willingly allow them to develop a sense of self-entitlement and lack of respect for authority. In that case, we are not showing love, as we facilitate and encourage behavior that will prevent them from developing into well-rounded adults.

Some parents result in yelling to correct the bad behavior. But shouting does not help at any stage during development. When tempers flare, and words are spouted out, there is no telling the damage they can cause.

Although the child needs to understand that what they just did is wrong, it does not help get angry. As parents, especially with strong-willed children, we must be in control of our emotions at all times.

Many parents get upset with toddlers who simply don't know any better because they have not learned the difference between right and wrong. This lack of emotional control will only exacerbate the situation.

Love is the ability to look past mistakes and guide your kid regardless of the emotional toll of doing so.

8

Love is tender and gentle even when gum gets stuck in their hair, and things are a bit messy. They have to learn somehow, and giving a child the proper space to learn makes a world of difference.

When counseling parents, I often tell them, love is the most powerful weapon you have as a parent. I have seen, so many children's lives are transformed when the parent simply starts to foster a greater sense of love in the home. When you create an environment of love, parenting will become easier.

They obey not because they are scared, but because they love you and want to make you happy.

A practical example I can give you on this is how I taught my child to clean her room. The frustration of coming home and seeing the place looking like a bomb was set off. As I said, yelling doesn't always work with strong-willed children, so I tried a different approach.

I said to my then 5-year-old, "Your room is messy again. Should we clean it up together before we make your bedtime hot chocolate?"

Then I proceeded to help clear up and turned it into a fun game. Soon she enjoyed clearing up so much she would ask if I wanted to help her clean-up. A few months after that, she would clean up all by herself and then shout, "Mom… dad, my room is clean… Can I have my cocoa now?"

But it gets better after six months of her newfound sense of accomplishment tidying up her room, and she started to observe when things were untidy in the house and ask why we hadn't cleaned up, mimicking my voice as best as she could.

The moral of the story is I replaced frustration with love; I was able to see things more objectively and help correct the undesirable behavior. I have seen others get the same results by replacing yelling with patience and love.

Guidance

It is often said that the first five years are the most formative of a child's life. It is the parent's responsibility to teach them and build up the child emotionally. When they have done a good deed and correct them when they have done something not so nice or pleasant, praise the child.

Guidance is more than teaching extremes or polar ends of morality. A recommendation is about helping them develop a moral compass, direction, and the noble traits and qualities we want them to have in life without indoctrinating them and stealing their ability to come to their conclusions.

A child does not understand the word "no," Unfortunately, one particular mention is the most familiar word a child will hear growing up.

During a child's exploration, a parent may look over to discover little Jane is digging in the dirt of a flowerpot. Of course, the mess is easy to fix, and the enjoyment of the soft, squishy ground between the fingers is new. However, it is the mess, not the action, that causes a resentful

"NO!" from the parent. It is not as if the parent doesn't want Jane to play in the dirt; it is the mess she is causing.

The child may not see the difference in playing with this sandbox inside the house to play outside. Yet, many parents may flare up and even spank the child as they lose emotional control. Understanding that your child does not understand the difference and taking the time to explain may be more beneficial than shouting at them in anger.

Many parent's sources of frustration stem from them repeating their lousy parenting habits and expecting different results. Yelling and spanking are not always effective and can serve only to re-enforce your child's strong will.

In situations like above, it would be wiser to remove the child from the sandbox outside and explain the difference. Redirection is one form of guidance. Although it is simple to remove the child and explain the difference between the sandbox and the flowerpot, there will be times when it is not so easy.

Security

One of the essential roles of a parent is to provide security. As our children are developing, it is our duty not only to guide them but also to protect them from harm. There are many dangers in the world they are growing up, particularly those brought about by the very choices our children may make.

11

But regardless of the source of danger, it is the parent's duty as a responsible adult to stand up for their child. If the child is bullied in school or feels pinned against various odds, it is the parent's job to fight for their child. These days, many parents leave the child to battle on their own with the mentality of the survival of the fittest. This mentality, however, may work in nature, but as humans, this concept is flawed. To build trust with a child, the parent must prove to the child that they will fight for them.

However, it is the parent's responsibility to provide the child with a safe environment free from verbal, emotional, and physical abuse. Even if that does mean taking away a new phone so that the texts stop, or the computer, so the hate mail ends.

Friendship

Inwardly most parents desire to be best friends with their kids. At one point in their lives, we may have been the center of their world, but kids will often become disinterested in their parents as time goes on.

This is why it is important where possible to foster friendship with our children at an early age. But the company with our children should not be used as an emotional crutch if we are unfulfilled in our own lives.

Becoming friends with our kids is about fostering a loving relationship, where the child knows we are their parent, but still feels they can talk to us, hang out with us or share with us without always having the obstacle of the type defined role of parenthood.

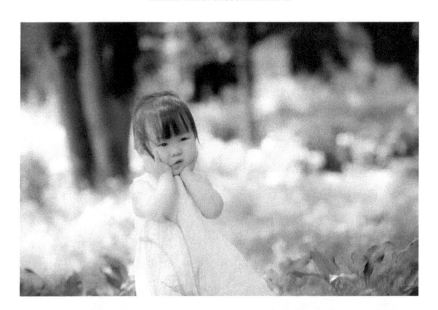

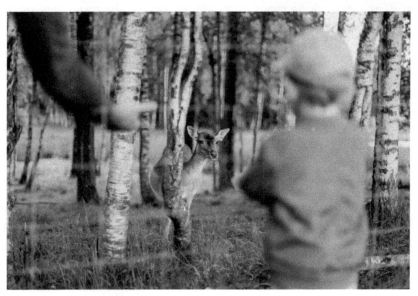

Chapter 2.

Positive Parenting Principles

Educating and disciplining children implies, among other things, establishing clear rules and limits. This is not always easy, even more so these days, but if parents adopt positive educational practices early on, it is possible to prevent future difficulties and problems. Cláudia Madeira Pereira, a clinical and health psychologist with a doctorate in clinical psychology, points out some acceptable practices that will make this task easier:

Talk to Your Child

Even if you are exhausted after a day at work, take some time out of your day to talk to your child. At dinner or before going to bed, ask him how his day was, using phrases such as "Tell me what you did today," "Tell me about the good things that happened today," or "Did something bad happen."

He can resort to several solutions. First, allow him to speak and listen to him without judgment or criticism. If you prefer, look for positive aspects that you can highlight and praise. Also, tell him about "what" and "how" to better deal with similar situations in the future.

14

Pay Attention to Good Behavior

Sometimes children learn that bad behavior is the best way to get parental attention... This is especially true for children whose parents pay attention to them only when they misbehave, even if that attention is negative, scolding them and rebuking them.

Promote Your Child's Autonomy and Responsibility

Some tasks, such as dressing in the morning, can be difficult for children. Even though it would be quicker for you to dress your child, you would prefer to encourage their autonomy and responsibility. Help your child by giving short and simple instructions on how to do the tasks.

To do this, use expressions such as "Take off your pajamas," "Now put on your shirt," or "Finally, put on your pants." Finish with a compliment, using phrases like "All right, you did a good job!" Sometimes it will not be enough to tell your child what to do; you may need to show him "what" and "how" to do it.

Establish Clear Rules

Be clear with your child about a set of rules. First, explain the direction succinctly and concretely. Second, make sure your child understands the direction and knows what is expected of him. In order for your child to be able to respect the rules more efficiently, try to give clear and straightforward directions, empathically, and positively.

You say like "It's time to go to bed. Let's go to the room now, and then I'll read you a story," usually work. It is common for children to challenge the rules in the early day,s but stay firm and consistent. Your child realizes that the new law is to be followed.

Set Limits

Try to be patient, and stand firm. Tell your child that an individual behavior must stop, explain the reasons, and inform him of the consequences of not obeying. In that case, preferably use phrases like "If you keep doing, then…" Immediately and consistently implement the products whenever lousy behavior occurs.

But do not resort to punishment or physical punishment (such as beating), as they only aggravate children's behavioral problems. Prefer to take a hobby or an object appreciated by your child for some time.

Stop the Tantrums

Try to ignore the tantrums, not paying attention to the child at such times. If possible, step back and pay attention to it only when the tantrums stop so that your child realizes that they can only get their attention when they stop throwing tantrums. At that point, prepare yourself, because your child will put him to the test.

At first, it is normal for tantrums to get worse. However, by systematically applying this method, the tantrums will eventually disappear.

You must be aware of your child's good behavior and value these behaviors whenever they occur, for example, by giving a compliment, a kiss, or a hug. If you do, the child will feel more accompanied.

Learn to Control Your Negative Feelings

There are times when any mother or father feels the nerves at the edge of the skin. Then try to do something to help him or her. You can, for example, listen to some music or take a few minutes of meditation. When you feel calmer, go back to your child and start again, using conciliatory phrasing in a sweet tone, like "I felt I did not know what to do, but I do know what to do with it now."

Have (A Lot Of) Patience

When you raise your child's communication (verbal and non-verbal) empathic and festive, it will contribute to a healthier and happier relationship between both. Educating and disciplining your child will require a great deal of your time and patience. No wonder they say being a mom and dad is tough, but it will be well worth it at them because it is the most rewarding job you can have.

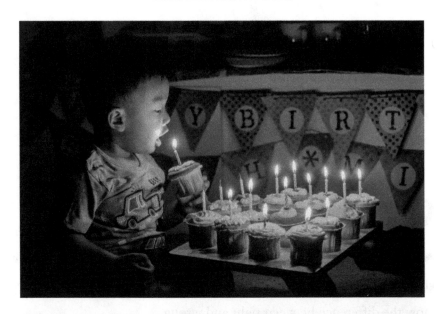

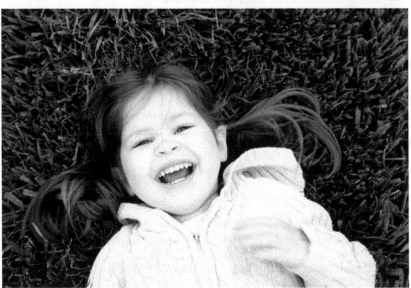

Chapter 3.

Parenting a Strong-Willed Child

Some toddlers can be difficult, and the need to train them comes in. We should not just claim that they would understand when they are grown, no. It may be too difficult for you to stop it when they are grown. They are toddlers, they are not dumb, and they know the difference between right and wrong.

Common Struggles Toddlers May Have

To begin, we need to understand why toddlers could be difficult. For the first time, they realize that they are separate individuals from their parents and caregivers. The initial thought is that he/she is part of the parent, but when they reach the toddler stage, they realize that this isn't true.

Furthermore, toddlers do not understand the logic of waiting and the logic behind having everything. They have no or little self-control, and in a nutshell, he/she may have a hard time balancing his/her needs with what you are providing as a parent or caregiver. Toddlers could be difficult; they could be funny too.

Here are four everyday situations your child could be struggling with:

1. He says no when he means yes. These happen when you are offering him a favorite treat.

2. He has a meltdown anytime you fail to understand his words.

3. He doesn't want any substitute. The blue pajamas or nothing else, even though they may not be washed or even after offering him the purple one.

4. He acts out when frustrated. Gives up everything when angry.

What is listed above are only acts which toddlers put on to manage strong feelings; since they are new to almost everything, they lack reasonable control over what controls them and how they can control it. They are toddlers; they soon find out that they have vocal powers, and that is when the crying, shouting, and yelling increases. They may also want to make different noises to see how they sound and the reactions of adults around them to such noise. They impulsively go into an activity without much or any thinking. They react differently to different situations; in fact, you can even place a tag around them. You can most often start with some funny names like bubbly, daredevil, determined, stubborn, cautious, adventurous, etc. It may beat you to know that some challenging toddler behavior is developmentally correct; they may be defiant, bossy, sassy, or impulsive. Still, they are just byproduct of what the child needs-independence.

Challenging Behaviors and Their Practical Solutions

Interrupting

Nothing can be so exasperating than a child who breaks in every time you are chatting with a friend. Toddlers don't interrupt with words all the time but their actions. And that is because they always seek attention from their parents and may be jealous if a friend or an adult is getting all of it. In this aspect, it is your fault. You can do the following:

- Chose the right locale for your meetings. A place where your child can enjoy while you talk with the adult. A park having a sandbox is something nice.

- Get a baby sitter. This would help a lot and would allow you to use all focus or concentration during the meeting. It is knowing that your child is in safe hands.

- Teach your children polite behavior. An excellent way to teach them is by reading them some books like The Bad Good Manners Book, by Babette Cole's Aliki's Manners, and What Do you Say Dear? By Style Joslin. Any book on good manners, you can lay your hands on. Could you read it to them every day?

- Schedule your phone calls. You wouldn't want your child to disturb you while you are on the market, so make the necessary preparations.

Lying

First, why do children lie? They have an active imagination, and they are very forgetful. These cute angels may also have what we call angel syndrome. A child who thinks that his parents believe he can do no wrong would do wrong on purpose. When asked, a lie comes to mind. Toddlers do lie, and it is natural for them to do so. How can you stop this?

- Always encourage truth-telling. You should not be angry at your child when he or she tells you the truth; instead, you should be happy. Show your child that honesty pays off.

- You should not accuse your child of any reason. Your comments, remarks should help your child not put him down.

- Don't weigh your child down with too many expectations. He or she would not understand. They are children, toddlers, not adults. You shouldn't be expecting too much from them.

- Build your trust. Assure your child that you trust him or her and don't puncture that trust.

Running Away

A running away toddler could be very funny. Like really? Where do they think they are going? But you have to be careful when this happens outdoors, especially on the walkway. Why do they run? Just like any other attitude displayed by a toddler, running away comes from a new sense of independence and the fact that he has legs that can run. You can't stop this; you can only control it:

- Stay close to them, and it should be okay for you to look ahead when they are running.

- Show him where he can run and where he can't. Allow him to explore the safe areas

- Entertain your child.

Tattling

Some of the time, kids tattle because they have not developed the social or emotional skills required to solve skills all by themselves. Tattling has a positive effect, too, and it means that your child is showing you that he/she understands the rules and knows right from wrong. Before we go too far, what is tattling? It means merely telling somebody, especially somebody in authority, about something terrible or somebody else's wrongdoing. Do you get a report from your child about everything? "Mom, Michael is playing in that person's car, Dad, Sarah is keeping a crayon in her pocket, Mom, Brian is playing with a sharp object... etc." That's tattling. The following steps can be taken:

- Assess the situation: Before you conclude that your child is a whiny tattletale, take stock of the problem.

- Put the work back on his shoulder for tattling. When your child understands that tattling only gets him more responsibility, he tends to mind his own business.

Teasing

You may agree, or not, teasing is just what life brings. It happens when it happens, and even toddlers are not left out of it. It is excruciating when toddlers are teased, and you should understand that as a parent. What can you do when a toddler is bullied? This may not work well for toddlers as they would require a verbal response.

- Your child should not respond. This could be hard, but it is a trick that can repel those guilty of the teasing offense.

- You can coach your child to "agree" with what the teaser is saying. He/she would look dumb when a child says, "I agree I suck my thumb."

- Ask for help. Your child can ask for help from anyone or any adult around.

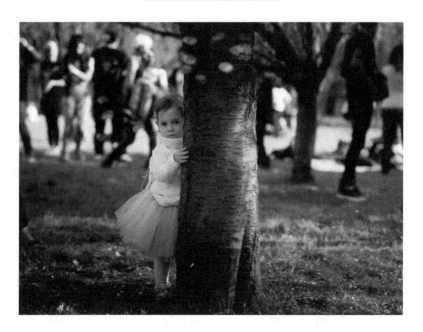

Chapter 4.

Managing Anger in Children

Mothers everywhere throughout the world have a difficult time dealing with their children. Regularly, they exclaim unnecessarily at children in their anger and loathe their activities from that point. Mothers try hard not to ruin their children's moods, but rather sometimes conditions outside anybody's ability to control show signs of mothers' improvement. They are unfit to endure the fiendishness and rebellion of their children. Indeed, even the best of mothers can lose their temper quickly.

The excitement of anger in you could be because of stress, budgetary issues, absence of adequate rest, appetite, or sickness. These variables repress you physically, and you show your failures as anger on your children.

Here are a couple of my proposals for you.

When you feel your anger is expanding alarmingly, move far from the scene. Practice some deep breathing and tallying exercises to cut down your tempers.

Return into your musings and tune in to what you said in your anger. This would doubtlessly not be your aim. Moreover, you might not want to set a case of a hollering mother to your children.

Practice how you will respond if your children make trouble. Practice out various circumstances and attempt to hold fast to these on certain occasions. This brings down the occurrence of anger.

Sometimes anger could be because of disappointment. You feel furious if children don't live and perform to your desires. You think to be a disappointment as a parent. Sometimes additionally, are the reason for your anger. Put aside a specific day or time of the week for yourself. Leave your children with your better half or another person and enjoy yourself. This could go about like an enormous destructor, and you can return revived entirely and brimming with vitality.

Anger is an emotion just like any other, which means that some people experience more of it than others do. The same is right for children. Sometimes your child will only be mad at you for no apparent reason, which can be very frustrating. A long time of constant disconnection and alienation from your child because of their anger will soon get you as angry as them or even more so.

Understanding your child's angry behaviors is the beginning of controlling your own anger because anger between children and parents is highly interconnected. We will look at some of the angry behaviors that children engage in and why they get angry, including the psychology of angry children and anger in different development stages.

Causes of Anger

As a parent, you keep up with your child's development and help them to grow holistically. Because children usually have not developed the full range of communication and self-expression tools that adults use to get their needs met, they tend to resort to anger to express their needs a lot of the time. When your baby was a toddler, your mother instincts would help you to interpret different angry cries accurately. However, as your child starts developing a whole life of its own with friends, school, and hobbies, you might find yourself falling short.

Hurt

This is the most common and universal cause of anger in children. Hardly any child will remain calm after getting hurt. Unless a child has been taught to suppress their pain by the parent, they are usually pretty honest in their expression of hurt. Everyday, things that might hurt a child include being neglected, the feelings of rejection, losing a friend, or feeling like their parents prefer a sibling over them.

Sadness

Children care a lot about the people and things around them because they make up their entire universe. The people in this universe include their playmates, parents, and close family. Things like school, the family house, and toys make up part of the universe. A child will be the saddest when this universe is threatened. A playmate moving away means that they will have either to play alone or find a new friend, which can be a terrifying experience. Other changes like separation and divorce, moving houses or school, or death are also very distressing.

Fear

Just like adults, children worry about their wellbeing and that of others. For example, some children get angry when they see their parents or loved ones struggling with an illness. In fact, a child is more likely to get angry when there is an ill family member than when they are sick themselves. Children of parents in dangerous careers like firefighters, the police, and soldiers also fear for the parent's safety, especially when they realize just how dangerous the job might be. For example, a child witnessing their father in a risky situation can get very upset and angry even if their job is reflected on television. The child might then withdraw and avoid the parent to try to protect themself from any possible future pain.

Frustrations

Children need to learn everything that adults take for granted, including movement, communication, and fine motor skills. They also need to watch as their bodies grow as they get older. At the same time, they will be comparing themselves to their peers in the house, at school, and in the playground. When a child lags in reaching some development milestone, it is widespread for them to get frustrated. The frustration manifests as anger and tends to last quite a long time.

Guilt

Children don't usually have the finely tuned range of emotions that adults have. So, when a child is feeling guilty for some mistake that they made, the first instinct is usually to lash out. Sometimes children will even feel guilty about problems they did not cause, such as a death or their parents divorcing. When you teach your child to do something and are unable to do it or forgets about it, this guilt will probably manifest as anger. This is especially tricky because you'll probably be angry at yourself. The way you handle such a situation affects the parental bond you form with your child as well as their emotional development.

ADHD

Children that have Attention Deficit Hyperactivity Disorder tend to have serious challenges in doing simple activities that other kids their age do with ease. The constant embarrassment and frustrations of performing worse than other children on ordinary tasks make them more likely to lash out and withdraw. The situation is worsened even further by parental frustrations and lack of compassion for their situation.

Embarrassment

A child who feels silly or awkward in a social situation and a child who just performed severely in a baseball game is likely to react the same way—by getting angry. Some children get angry when they are embarrassed and might even cry or hit whatever is closest to them. The

30

fear of being judged makes them lash out in anger to distract themselves from their disappointment with their own behavior.

Angry Behaviors

Children display their anger in different ways. Some of the ways that children express anger can be interpreted as normal child behaviors, which is why some parents overlook them and fail to look for the underlying cause of irritation. It's useful to recognize anger in your kid while still young, and they have not learned to mask the rage or hide it entirely from you. The sooner you find the underlying cause of angry behaviors, the easier it will be to solve the underlying problem. It's also essential that you deal with your child's anger issues appropriately.

Overreacting to an episode of anger might give your child the wrong idea about expressing anger. It's when your child forms a pattern of angry behaviors that you should be concerned. However, severe, isolated incidences are usually a pure expression of anger by a child who does not know how to express their anger. Take these moments as teachable moments and teach your child to express their anger correctly.

Children develop anger management issues when they suppress emotions like grief, fear, and hurt. The vulnerability that these feelings bring terrifies a kid and makes them defensive. This defensiveness makes children defiant, even cruel. Everything a child does to suppress exposure will always be intended to assert their independence. While they are locking you away to show you that they do not need you, it is just a disguised cry for help.

Withdrawal

Sometimes a child just wants to talk to their dolls or be alone, which is perfectly normal. Assuming a child is enjoying their own company, lonesomeness isn't a problem. It becomes a problem when your child stays alone, but does not seem to be enjoying it and is sad. Kids who feel like their problems aren't recognized or appreciated by their caregivers tend to express their anger by withdrawing. A child will express reluctance to family activities, spend a lot of time alone, and lock themselves in rooms like the bathroom or their bedroom alone. A child who does not have many friends and plays alone might be dealing with some serious anger issues and intervention.

Temper Tantrums

A two-year-old child with a temper tantrum where they kick and hits on everything in sight because you did not buy them or toy, they wanted at the mall is quite common. This is a widespread habit of children in the terrible twos. It is when your nine-year-old does something like that, you should be worried. Generally, you must see an improvement in your child's ability to handle disappointments when things don't go their way. It's just a part of the growth in their emotional and behavioral capabilities.

Irritability/Impatience

An impatient child wants to get what they want "right now!" and not a second later. They will make a fuss and become irritable at any time there is a delay. This goes for anything from a juice box coming out of the fridge to getting a toy delivered after buying it online. Irritability usually shows frustrations in other areas of life, such as reaching development milestones. The irritability will probably continue until they get to the same level as their peers unless you intercede and help them resolve the frustration.

Aggression

Aggression in children is usually a sign of anger at the most distressing levels. With violent behavior, the child is generally feeling pretty helpless and vulnerable. And along with violent behavior like kicking and biting, you'll start to see them engaging in destructive behaviors. This includes smashing toys, tearing books, and chucking away food (often at other people's heads). Destruction of property is usually the loudest cry for help and indicates that your child needs exceptional service, especially when the behavior is consistent and intentional.

Fighting and bullying

The occasional skirmish over a swing at the playground can merely be a sign of a strong-willed or dominant kid. As long as you teach them to be more aware of other kids' needs, there should be no trouble there. What you should look out for is a growing habit of getting into confrontations with other children. Especially worrisome is a child picking fights with older children. It's usually an indication that children want to prove themselves, often due to frustrations in attaining developmental milestones.

Insults and Bad Language

When you don't teach your child to handle their anger constructively, it will likely burst through the surface with explosive insults. When anger episode remains unresolved for a long time, the occasional insult gives way to foul language that usually comes in explosive outbursts. Children raised by angry parents often notice and adopt their parents' habits, such as insulting others and cussing. However, the insults and cussing are usually a veneer to cover up their fears and very often self-blame for the strife around the house. In the early teenage years, children will have started to model their parents' behaviors, including physical violence and drug use, due to a difficult home situation's frustrations.

Hurting Animals and Other Children

Children are usually very gentle with animals like pets. Any form of cruelty, like hurting an animal, shows that a child has some unexpressed anger that they are repressing. In many cases, seeking to hurt an innocent animal, as well as nastiness towards a younger sibling, indicates that a child may have been or felt abused. It's a way of paying back a physical assault in kind.

Reflexive Opposition

When children are angry with their parents, they are more likely to refuse to follow instructions out of spite. Children get hostile when they are angry at some unfairness that they cannot do anything about. The only way to even out the score becomes rebellion. The same goes for vengefulness. A child who is continuously seeking revenge against people who wrong them (peers or adults) is usually fighting back against the anger they feel for being misunderstood or a parent treating them with no compassion. This is very common for children who have grown up under a strict parent and received disciplinary action for every mistake they made.

Blaming Others for Mess-ups

A child who is always blaming others for mistakes is usually hiding their anger at having disappointed themselves. The fear of consequences for errors might also cause it.

How to Deal With an Angry Child

Parental anger management goes beyond improving your wellbeing as a parent. As crucial as parental wellbeing is, it does not make up for being clueless about how you're supposed to handle your angry child. Parental and child anger are intertwined.

If your child is angry, they are likely to pass the anger on to you with their actions. And when you're angry, you'll probably do something to anger your child like screaming at them In this section; we will cover the practical strategies that you can apply in dealing with your angry child.

Delay

This is the most critical lesson in handling your anger. Delay your anger for as long as possible regardless of the mistake that your child made. For example, if you are picking them up from mall jail, delay the confrontation until you get in the car, then until you get home, and then after a time-out in their room. You get around to addressing the issue at hand, and you'll have calmed down enough to have a clear head for problem-solving.

Breathing Exercises

Take a few calming breaths before dealing with any child-related stress. This allows you to quiet down your anxiety and stay grounded. Only then can you manage trying moments with your kids gracefully and calmly.

Recreation

Sometimes all you need to keep your child happy is some happy moments. When you engage in entertainment such as sports with your child, the physical activity acts as a salve to anger and allows both of you to release the frustrations trapped deep within. The time you spend together in play strengthens your connection to your child and facilitates some healthy communication.

Teaching Self-expression

Children express a range of emotions like fear, worry, embarrassment, and sadness, among others, with anger. For a toddler who cannot speak, this may be acceptable. As your child grows and learns to talk, you should teach them how to express their needs, fears, and worries. Question your child about his or her feelings when they are upset so that you can become more adept at interpreting their frustrations. A good sense of self-expression will help your child talk about issues that bother them instead of getting angry.

Healthy Communication

Sometimes a child will get angry because they need to feel heard and seen, and they aren't getting that from the world. If your child is doing something, you should be the greatest fan. When you're a parent, communication with your child goes beyond words. Children communicate with their body language, their actions, and their performance in school. It is your place to decode everything your child is telling you and move to fulfill their needs.

Understanding/Relating

When you capture your child doing something naughty in the spur of the moment, your own adult interpretation of right and wrong tends to take over and override your ability to relate. For example, a two-year-old child would not have the smarts to know that flour isn't something to play with. It would be best if you always tried to look at a situation from your child's perspective before handing out your punishment.

Listening

Parents with naughty kids tend to have a lot more trouble with this particular strategy. You assume that your child did it even before you know the situation just because they have given you so much grief in the past. What this does is that it makes your child feel like you don't believe in them that you are not on their side. Who knows, maybe your daughter or son's impossible explanation will crack you up and bring some comic relief to a tense situation.

Forgive

Sometimes it helps to react with compassion in place of anger, especially when you have been interacting with your child through anger a lot. For example, when you need to teach an important life lesson that might help your child change their behavior, you can get a lot further over an ice cream than screaming at them across the room.

Be the Parent

The role of a parent entails providing, protecting, and guiding. It's the same even when you have caught your child in a mess-up. It would be greatest if you were more mature and more levelheaded so that you can solve the problem at hand. Sometimes your child is only acting out because they lack the knowledge to deal with their personal issues. You should offer guidance on how to do so or find a mentor if you are unqualified to deal with a problem. Finally, it would help if you were a role model for your child in everything that you do. If you don't know how to hold your anger or if your life isn't organized, your child will probably mirror that.

Chapter 5.

No More Yelling

(How to Teach Without Yelling)

Why do we yell at our children? We love our children; we do not want any harm to come to them; we do not want to see them cry, and we never want to see them upset; yet, we yell.

Most parents yell at their children for one of a few reasons. The first reason is the most obvious; the parents yell at their children because they feel they have run out of options. They think that the discipline has not worked; talking to the child has not worked; that pleading and bribing the child has not worked. Therefore, they resort to yelling.

The second reason that the parents yell is that they do not know how to parent any other way. Most of the time, the parents that yell were yelled at when they were children. It is simply passed from one generation to the next, and the parent does not know how to break the cycle.

The third reason parents yell has nothing to do with the child, but it is simply because they have allowed themselves to become overwhelmed with life. They feel that they're not being heard, not only when it comes to their children but also in life. They may have taken more than they can handle, and, as a result, they end up feeling emotionally charged all of the time. Because these parents do not know how to deal with their emotions, they end up yelling at their kids, even when their child makes the slightest mistake.

What happens when we yell at our children? Studies have shown that yelling at our children has the same effect on them as spanking and that yelling has psychological consequences that can last long into the future. When we yell at our children, we are changing the way that their brain works. Yelling is nothing more than another form of abuse, and it affects the child's mind in the same way as physical abuse does. Yelling can increase a child's risk of developing depression, mental disorders, and personality disorders; it can also increase the risk of suicide and decrease brain activity.

When a child is yelled at by the parent, they learn that they should be afraid of the parent instead of trusting them. This means that the child will be less likely to try and please the parent, which usually will cause the parent to become more upset and yell even more. Meaning that the children will have a hard time trusting others as they grow and will have a hard time feeling secure as adults. Yelling can also lead to anxiety issues as the child grows.

When a parent yells at a child, the child quickly learns that it is easier to tune the adult out than to listen to the constant yelling. This, of course, causes the adult to become even more upset because the child still is not doing what they requested, and it causes even a more significant divide between the parent and child.

As I stated earlier, there is never any reason for you to cause damage to your relationship with your child. There is nothing so severe that your child could do that it would be appropriate for you to generate the child not to trust you.

You have to remember that you are your child's safe place. You are the one person that they are supposed to be able to turn to, no matter who turns against them or what is going on in their lives. You are their entire world, and they want you to continue being so. Yelling at your child shows them that they are not even safe when they are with you, and it will not produce a well-balanced child as they grow older.

What are you as the parent supposed to do? You have to learn alternatives to yelling. You can do many things instead of yelling at your child, but before we get into those, I want to take a few minutes to talk about your life in general.

Most parents yell at their children because their own life is out of control. You have to get your life under control, and you have to do it NOW. Make sure that you take the steps that you need to take to reduce the stress in your life, get your budget under control, and make sure that you are getting done everything you need to get done daily.

Once you have your life figured out, it is time to start changing your behavior. Yes, it is time to focus on how you behave instead of how your child is behaving.

Taking deep breaths is a great way to calm yourself and stop yourself from yelling at your child. Close your eyes and inhale through your nose, hold the breath for a few seconds, and exhale through your mouth. Really think about what is going on. Is it really the child that you are upset with, or are you just upset in general?

Calmly address the behavior. Just because you cannot yell at your kids does not mean that you cannot address lousy behavior and get them to understand that it is unacceptable. For example, if you have a hard time getting your toddler to pick up their toys after they are done playing with them, calmly tell the toddler that if they do not pick up the toys, you are going to take them away. Give them a few minutes to pick up their toys, and if the toys are not put away, calmly bag up the toys and take them out. Allow the toddler to earn the toys back through good behavior.

See how simple that was? You taught your toddler a lesson, the boys got cleaned up, and you did not have to yell your head off and scare your toddler half to death.

We have been taught that punishment is a teaching tool when, in reality, it is merely a way to cause pain in one way or another. A teaching tool is a discipline, which is ultimately the opposite of punishment. Take a few moments to look at the situation and think about how you can teach your toddler what you want them to do and how you can ensure that they do it in the future. Then make sure that you follow through every single time.

Instead of yelling, use a firm but calm voice. Trust me, and nothing will tell your toddler that you mean business other than a quiet, firm agent. Keep your voice low so that your child has to pay attention to hear from you and make them work to listen to what you are saying. The calmer that you can stay, the more impact your words will make, and the more attention your child will pay to what you are saying.

Before you begin screaming at your child because they have misbehaved, take a few minutes to figure out why the toddler has misbehaved. This is something that I have tried to focus on throughout this book because, as adults, it is so easy for us to forget that toddlers usually have a reason for misbehaving. It has nothing to do with breaking the rules or upsetting you. Generally, when a toddler misbehaves, they need something, whether it be food, a nap, or time away from an individual situation.

Follow through instead of nagging and then yelling. If you tell your children to turn off the television and you come back five minutes later to a child still watching television, walk up, turn off the television, and redirect your child. So much yelling could be avoided if parents followed through and stopped what I call lazy parenting.

Lazy parenting is talking simply to hear their own voice, knowing that what they are requesting is not going to be done, threatening the child without following through, and then screaming in anger when the child does not do as asked. Don't practice lazy parenting.

If you find that your child cannot do the tasks you are requesting of him or her, you need to adjust your expectations instead of screaming your head off. For example, my youngest son suffers from ADHD, as well as a few other issues. This means that while I can tell to his sister—who is only 1 year older than him—to go clean her room and she is able to do it, I have to break the tasks down for him, telling him each step, one at a time as he completes the one before. I had to change my expectations because telling him to clean his room usually meant that he went to his place, sat on his bed, and looked around wholly overwhelmed with the task.

Remember that each child is different, and while one child may be able to do one task, it may be more challenging for the next child, and you might have to adjust your expectations, which is still much more straightforward than yelling at your child.

Chapter 6.

Calm and Confident Leader

So much of disciplining toddlers lovingly and respectfully depends on this energy, that of a calm and confident leader. Toddlers look to their parents for successful cues on how they should proceed in the world, and modeling is the most effective way to show them what is expected of them.

In all of your interactions with your toddler moving forward, remember this. You can and should respectfully acknowledge their fears, frustrations, issues, and upsets, but you should do this as the calm and confident leader they need. In doing so, you set the alarm for both their success and yours.

Your Child is Afraid

Anxiety is one of the major problems most parents face during potty-training, which can be very crippling. The child may be suffering from general anxiety, reflecting on the potty-training process or suffering from potty-training anxiety. Either way, it is important to face this problem head-on, as you won't be able to get anything done if your child is afraid.

First, you should identify the type of anxiety your child suffers from. If the child suffers from general anxiety, you can visit a therapist for diagnosis and treatment. There is a condition known as a generalized anxiety disorder in which the kid worries about a variety of issues, which should not be a source of worry normally. Below is an excerpt from a Boston Children's Hospital publication describing the condition.

Fear can make the child refuse to sit on a potty or toilet. Some children even get scared of making a bowel movement in the potty while some may be afraid of the toilet flushing. Anxiety can also cause the child to wet themselves or defecate in places you don't expect.

If the child is afraid of sitting on the potty or pooping in the potty chair, you should start by encouraging the child to sit on the potty periodically with clothes on at first, then with clothes off later. You can get them accustomed to the potty by decorating it with stickers together and getting toys which, the child can only play with when he sits on the potty. Make sure the potty is comfortable enough for the child. To help with this, let the child join you in shopping for the potty before you start potty-training. You should then pick the one the child chooses.

The child has an accident while playing.

It is common for a child to wet or soil themselves while playing, usually due to excitement or distraction. First, you should make sure it isn't due to a medical issue such as incontinence or an overactive bladder.

Generally, children are not able to control their bladder until around the age of three or four. Even at that age, accidents are still common, especially during the night. The digestive tract has nerves which can be triggered by an emotional, exciting, or stressful event.

The child may get carried away playing and ignore the urge to ease themselves until it becomes uncontrollable or may simply wet themselves due to too much excitement or stimulation. To prevent this, you should help the child follow a consistent bathroom routine and make sure they ease themselves before going out to play.

Potty accidents when playing could also be caused by constipation or by the child holding it in deliberately. The child may choose to hold it in, either as a result of an emotional reaction or anxiety. However, accidents may then happen during play as the child gets too relaxed or too excited to control their bladder or bowel. When this happens, do not ignore the situation or yell at the child. Let the child calm down first and then proceed to clean the mess together. The child shouldn't return to playing until he has been cleaned up and the mess disposed of properly.

While the child is playing, you can also make them take short breaks to go to the bathroom. This will help in emptying his bladder and bowels and also to calm him down. You also can limit any adrenaline-inducing play for the meantime. Things such as throwing the child up or swinging them around can cause an adrenaline spike or a bit of fear, thereby making the child lose control of their bowels and bladder.

Though potty accidents can be frustrating, you should keep in mind that accidents while playing are normal during potty-training and result from a natural response to excitement or anxiety. Since the child is still developing, issues such as this may occur frequently, but the child should grow out of it with age. However, if this gets too severe or continues till over the age of five, it is advisable to visit a medical professional.

Your son/daughter doesn't want to go to the bathroom with you.

Your child may refuse to go to the bathroom with you or anyone else present. This isn't unusual. Children start to develop a sense of awareness at a period, and they start being conscious of their bodies. The child may refuse to go to the bathroom with you or anyone to show independence. You must, therefore, be prepared to handle this carefully as a parent.

Leaving the child unsupervised, in this case, will lead to lots of cleaning for you. They have to learn how to use the potty or toilet, wipe themselves and flush, and wash their hands. If they learn how to do these correctly, they'll have the freedom to use the bathroom on their own.

From another perspective, your child may be self-conscious or ashamed of his body. You should check for any sign of abuse, either physical or emotional. A child getting ashamed of his or her body suddenly may be a sign of abuse. Do visit a therapist if the child's behavior gets suspicious.

Do not make fun of any of his physical attributes. This can affect the child's self-esteem negatively. If the child is uncomfortable with you being with him or her in the bathroom, you can ask a family member of the same gender to accompany them.

The child may refuse your company in the bathroom also as a way of showing independence. This is okay, but you should make sure he or she has learned the process correctly. Let them recite the steps to take until you are satisfied. You can remind them of what he or she should do while they are inside to be safe. Pediatric psychologists have explained that it is vital for the child to create boundaries around their bodies as they start gaining independence and self-awareness.

Respecting your child's boundaries will go a long way in creating a sense of self-respect and improving the child's self-esteem. This will also teach the child to respect other people's boundaries as children learn through imitation. However, you should teach the child to be open with you and to feel free to talk about any issue.

The Child Poops Next to the Potty

You may have gotten your child to stop going in his or her underwear, but you may be faced with another problem—the child misses when he or she tries to poop in the potty or poops next to it instead. To stop this, you should first observe the child to determine why he does it. So you have to get the specific cause. From my experience as a parent, I'll list the primary reasons why a child "misses" or may poop next to the potty deliberately.

First, you may have trained your child to stop using diapers or going in their underwear, but the child may not be used to the potty yet. They know they shouldn't poop in their underwear, but may be scared of using the potty. They then choose to poop next to the potty instead. That is why it's essential to get your child familiar with the potty chair as soon as you start potty-training.

Please encourage them to sit on the potty at frequent intervals and make sure they are comfortable sitting on the potty. You can motivate with toys and children's books. Praise them if they eventually poop inside the potty. If accidents occur, clean up the mess and let them see you put it inside the potty. They'll finally learn that poop should always go in the potty.

Also, if the potty isn't easily accessible, accidents may happen. Children have a hard time correctly recognizing the urge to go beforehand, so they may be hard-pressed before he eventually decides to use the potty. However, if they can't get to the potty on time, they may no longer be able to hold it in, thereby causing them to poop close to the potty instead. You should make sure that the potty chair is placed where the child can reach it easily. After getting a suitable location, make sure the potty is placed there consistently.

As we've said many times, you should make sure your child's underwear and clothes are easily removable. This will help your child hop into the potty on time as precious time won't be wasted on trying to get his clothes off. If it's too late for the child to hold it in, he may poop just before he sits on the potty.

Don't get worked up if he poops next to the potty instead of in it. When this happens, calmly correct them and motivate them to do better next time. Let him or her know you; we appreciate their effort in trying to use the potty instead of going in his underwear. Be patient with the child. Potty-training doesn't last forever, and you'll be over it in no time.

The Child is Very Stubborn

A stubborn child can seem impossible to potty train, and you may run out of options quickly as the child continues being headstrong. The child may counter every instruction you give him with a strong "No" and only accepts things on his terms. How then do you potty train such a child? You might be tempted to yell, spank the child, or punish him some other way. Potty-training, which should be fun for the child, now becomes a power tussle each day.

You should save yourself the stress of potty-training a child that isn't ready. If you decide to wait until the child is ready, in the meantime, you can prepare the child through some methods. You can get fun potty-training books or videos made for children.

Even when the child is ready for potty-training, you may still encounter some resistance. First, you should get rid of all the diapers in the house. Let the child be aware of this and calmly tell him diapers are no longer an option. With no other choice, the child will eventually cooperate.

If the child firmly refuses to sit on the potty, do not try to force him physically. If you do this, he will eventually develop an aversion toward the potty. It would also be best if you didn't get into a screaming match with the child when he refuses to sit. It's your job as an adult to manage the situation calmly. Motivate them with words instead.

You can also create an illusion of choice for the child. For example, you can say, "Will you sit on the potty or on the toilet seat?" The child will be happy to get to choose themselves and will then select one of the options. Get the child used to the process gradually instead of trying everything at once.

However, it would be best if you were firm with your instructions and demands. Repeat them until the child eventually uses the potty or sits on the toilet. Do not bribe the child or let them manipulate you; this will only make the situation worse.

My Child Wets the Bed

Nighttime continence takes time. Even if your child has been toilet-trained for weeks, months, or even years, accidents will happen. But don't fret. A useful technique that is highly recommended is the 'last-minute pee.' This means before going to bed, and your child should use the bathroom. As the name suggests, this should be at the very last minute before they are getting into bed. This is often all it takes to help a child stay dry at night. Also, make sure you have a waterproof sheet protecting their mattress and consider investing in some nighttime diapers if you have exhausted the other options.

My Child has Autism

Autism, or autism spectrum disorders (ASD) need not be a barrier to potty-training, provided you heed the advice given throughout this book. Bear in mind that you should only potty train when your child is ready. Even if your child is still in diapers longer than other kids, don't worry. It's not a race.

Potty-training will also take a little longer for ASD kids, so be patient. Use your knowledge of your child's quirks to help the potty-training process. For example, if the diaper-free sensation is quite unbearable for your child, consider cutting a hole in the bottom of it.

Use the power of routine to familiarize your child with the toilet process and do everything in the exact same order.

It's useful to use visual cues to really cement this routine—create a poster or flow-chart to demonstrate what happens when you use a potty. Include things like "Johnny needs to do a pee" right up until "Johnny washes his hands." Get a few copies and place one in the bathroom, which can be easily seen, and another in another highly visible part of the house. Talk about it often and refer to the poster. It can also help your child draw accompanying pictures—this very action will often help to cement notions about the potty in their brain.

Use environmental cues to comfort your child: ensure that the bathroom is calm, peaceful, and quiet. Use lighting to add to the sense of calm, and consider placing the potty somewhere private for your child.

The child follows the potty routine at home but not at the daycare.

You may be fully satisfied with your child's potty-training progress at home, but the child doesn't follow the daycare routine. It may even look as if the child has never been introduced to potty-training. The first thing you should do is to find out the actual cause. I'll help explain some of the possible causes with the appropriate solutions just below.

First, the issue may be due to the changing of environment. The child might be used to the potty or toilet at home, his books and toys, and your ever-present self. The daycare might be a whole new experience for the child, with strange faces, different facilities, and the many other kids present too. The child may also not be able to follow the usual bathroom routine at the normal time he does while at home. All these can be very confusing and destabilizing for the child.

To help the child overcome this, you can meet with the provider to help make some adjustments to the potty routine at the daycare for your child. If the daycare provider permits, you can bring along the child's home potty and toys to give them a familiar feeling. Also, inform the provider about your child's current level of progress. The child shouldn't be placed on a toilet seat if he has just started using the potty. The provider should stick with what the child is capable of.

Also, a shy child might not speak up if he has to use the bathroom, mostly if the daycare is filled with unfamiliar faces. The child may not want these strange caregivers to see them naked. To help with this, meet with the caregiver in charge of your child and introduce them. Let the child get comfortable with them and tell them they are free to call for the caregiver if they need anything. You can also implore the caregiver to pay extra attention to your child.

At the daycare, the child may be around children who haven't been potty trained yet. Surrounded by diapers, your child may be tempted or influenced to go in his or her underwear to be like the other children. To prevent regression, you can meet the caregiver to come up with a suitable solution together. The child can either be grouped with other potty-trained children, or you can make a copy of the child's bathroom routine at home, which would be given to the caregiver. The caregiver can then make sure the child follows this routine carefully.

You should also request reports from the daycare periodically to know about the child's progress. You should reward the child whenever they have a dry day and motivate them if accidents happen.

You've tried to potty train the child previously and failed. How do you start over again?

First, starting potty-training when the child isn't ready is one of the most common reasons for potty-training failure. A toddler who is not physically and mentally prepared for potty-training will have a hard time learning the process. This time around, you should make sure the child is fully prepared for potty-training. You can take a little time before you start potty-training again after the previous failure.

Also, switching to using diapers once you get tired of cleaning up is sure to fail at potty-training. Lack of consistency is part of the common reason parents fail at potty-training. When you get ready to start afresh, you must be prepared to spend a whole lot of time on the process. Choose a period when you'll be completely available. You should follow consistent bathroom routines and potty rituals this time around.

Another reason you may fail at potty-training is if you make the process as a strict and serious one. If you force the child to do your bidding each time or punish the child whenever accidents happen, the child will not gain the necessary confidence to develop bathroom independence. Potty-training should be a fun and rewarding experience for you and the child. Make sure to get toys, stickers, and training products suited for the child this time around.

You might need to switch from the previous methods you used or make them more fun. Be ready to learn together with the child this time around. It would be best if you also let the child be involved in the process. You can give them simple chores such as getting the soap or toilet paper, or any other simple task. Reward the child when he completes these tasks successfully.

Let the child know in advance that you are about to resume potty-training. Make the process sound exciting for the child to make them more enthusiastic. Also, as a parent, make up your mind to complete the process this time around.

The child holds it in and refuses to go to the toilet.

According to North Fulton Pediatrics, more than five percent of children refuse potty-training. To overcome this, you have to look for the root cause of the problem—why the child has refused to poop.

Refusing to poop might result from anxiety, or the child may be scared of sitting on the potty or the toilet. When you then stop using diapers at the start of potty-training, the child is now left with no choice but to hold it in as a result of fear. It has also been suggested that holding it in might be a reaction to a bad experience with pooping. For example, when the child has suffered from constipation or other bowel issues and has gone through a painful bowel movement, he may associate the succeeding bowel movements with that memory.

The child may just refuse to poop as a way of rejecting potty-training. The child may refuse your instructions and prefer to hold it in instead as an act of defiance.

Stool withholding can also be caused by constipation itself. The child may continue to withhold stool if he finds bowel movement difficult. The more the child withholds, the worse it becomes as stool starts getting compacted in the child's colon. Watery stool eventually leaks out without the child being able to control it. The muscles that control bowel movements might also be affected.

Forcing the child to poop won't work in correcting this, but there are practical ways you can get the child to resume normal bowel habits. If the stool withholding is a result of anxiety, continuously reassure the child and make them comfortable. A child needs to be relaxed to have a smooth bowel movement. Some children are scared of pooping in the potty or toilet as they see the poop as a part of themselves. You should explain to such a kid that poop needs to go to the bathroom to stay healthy.

Let the child talk about his worries, and while you reassure them, help and face them too. For example, if the child is scared of the toilet, you can sit on the toilet in front of them to assure or encourage them to sit while you hold them.

If the child withholds stool as a way of avoiding potty-training, carefully explain why he needs to go and look for ways to make potty-training fun for the child. Do not place pressure on them to use the toilet. After that, stop talking about the issue.

If the stool withholding is due to constipation, you can make some changes to the child's diet. Also, increase his fluid intake if necessary. A medical professional may also prescribe stool softeners or mild laxatives to get the child to release his bowels.

Chapter 7.

Common Parenting Mistakes When Training Toddlers

I t is introduced to some of the mistakes parents make when training their little children. If you find yourself susceptible to any of these mistakes, you should navigate them with better strategies founded on a basic principle shown in the latter part of this study guide.

Distorting the Routine

Toddlers work at their best capacities when the routine is predictable. Whether it is sleep, food, or alertness, you have to know your toddlers' daily activities and make them repetitive. Some parents don't know the circadian rhythm of their toddlers. This is the internal clock in the brain of a person. It measures the consistencies in the sleepiness and activeness of a person at regular intervals. As a parent, you should monitor the characters in the sleep- and wake-cycle of your toddler, as well as yours.

Using a Method of Coercion

One of the parental attitudes that experts sorely disapprove of is one in which the parent pressures or coerces toddlers into doing an action. It doesn't matter whether your toddler's activity is coerced into doing is wrong or not; pressuring your toddlers is a vice that has lifetime detriments on them. Coercion has terrible effects on your toddler's eating attitude.

Modest Method of Coercion Bribery

Smart parents find a way around things. This is detrimental to the toddler's behavior. They often apply a subtle coercion method by promising the toddler a reward of a favorite food after eating a disliked food. According to psychologist Dr. Leann Birch of the Pennsylvania State University, if the promised food is dessert, it makes the toddler value dessert more than more nutritious foods like vegetables and meats.

Serving Toddlers Big Food Items

According to the American Dietetic Association in Chicago, parents tend to serve children's food items that are not compatible with their stomachs. When the food is relatively significant to the child, they feel intimidated and frustrated to complete a considerable meal's seemingly massive task.

Succumbing to Your Toddler's Denial of New Foods

This should not be mistaken for coercion. It merely means some parents make the mistake of not trying the law of consistency when introducing new foods to their toddlers.

As Dr. Birch notes, it may require between 10 to 15 times of presentation before a toddler can finally adopt a new food. Dr. Jean Skinner, another reputable dietitian at the University of Tennessee, also posits that to fulfill the necessary criterion of your toddlers eating a variety of foods, you need to offer a variety of foods consistently.

According to Satter, a display of hysterical happiness when the toddler finally accepts to eat a new food may also make the child avoid the food eventually.

Intolerance to Messy Mealtimes

Excessiveness is when you expect a toddler to keep all the table manners you have acquired in the social world. Many parents think the taste is the only way food is enjoyed. While this is true for an adult, it isn't the case for a toddler. According to experts in Food and Nutrition Science, children use many sensory organs to enjoy food. They tend to enjoy the food more when they play with it and get themselves all messy.

Many parents who express sore displeasure to these messy eating manners have the tendency to distort the enjoyment toddlers have when eating. For children, forget about table manners and let them eat. The nutrition they consume takes more importance than whether they eat neatly or not. Having seen some of the mistakes that parents make when training toddlers, it is also beneficial to see some general consequences.

Rigidly Rebuking Your Toddler's Mistakes

Correcting mistakes that are made is necessary, but when the scrutiny becomes intense, you may be digging a very deep pitfall for your toddlers in the future. Parents who take an extreme disciplinary approach to their children's mistakes usually have the conception that this will make them better and perfect.

When the kid eventually grows into an adult and makes mistakes, their sense of personal worth takes a dent. They punish themselves by subjecting their-self to self-flagellating thoughts, which is a gateway to depression. They take a rigid approach to correct themselves. In extreme cases, they may resort to self-harm. Other significant areas where parents often make mistakes are eating habits and toilet manners.

Chapter 8.

Children Discipline - Parenting Tips

Taking a solid stand is anything but an awful thing for most guardians to learn. Children need discipline. It shows them what is proper conduct - and what isn't. Some of the time, training is vital to teaching children results. Keep it brief, short, and regard the youngster's sentiments. Being exacting doesn't mean manhandling a tyke or deprecating them. It implies leading the pack to show them the proper behavior in a legitimate, aware, and safe way.

For such a large number of guardians, a dread of squashing a youngster's soul, or overpowering them with an excessive amount of cutoff points, make them take a rearward sitting arrangement on the order train, just to be looked with bratty, wild, and impolite children for a considerable length of time to come.

Children do not just need limits; they need them. It makes them feel safe, and indeed, even cherished. They haven't correctly figured out how to control their inclinations and wants yet, and look to you, the parent, as a manual for demonstrating to them what conduct is all right and what isn't. The order is more than an apparatus for creating respectful children - it's a device to creating balanced and genuinely sound children.

Picking the correct type of order might be one of the hardest things a parent needs to do. Each youngster is extraordinary, and keeping in mind that breaks may work superbly with one another may require a light tap on the behind occasionally to express what is on your account. Follow these essential hints from youngster advancement master T. Berry Brazelton, M.D.

Consider a Child's Stage of Development

Knowing why your little child keeps on playing in the can even after you've disclosed to them no multiple times may enable you to all the more likely arrangement with your disappointments and make sense of if your tyke is, in reality, being disobedient, or merely investigating their existence in a typical and healthy way.

Fit the Discipline to the Child's State of Development

Babies can frequently be occupied absent much flourish, while more seasoned children may require a break or other type of control to get them to stop what they're doing. Make sense of what works best for each phase of a tyke's development for better outcomes.

Pick Discipline That Fits the Child

All you needed to do was shake your head at my girl in objection, and she'd started sobbing uncontrollably and stop what she was doing. Not so with my child. He once stressed that his conduct would offend you,

TIPS AND TRICKS FOR GOOD PARENTING

so he needs a more vigorous style to train him directly from off-base. Try not to utilize a similar form of control for each youngster. The chances are it'll work for a few and nobody else.

Be a Good Role Model

When your tyke sees you lose your temper when you don't get your specific manner, think about what, they'll do likewise. Tell your children the best way to deal with dissatisfaction and disappointment by being a good role model.

Continuously Show Children Love and Tenderness

At the point when the Discipline Is Over. Regardless of whether it's time alone in their room or tap on the hand, dependably embrace your kid and strengthen the way that you adore them, notwithstanding when they resist. It's comforting to realize that you're still #1 in your parent's eyes - notwithstanding when you mess up.

While there are some substantial burdens to unforgiving physical discipline (forceful conduct, dread, slight), a few guardians have discovered that taking a stable remain (in a delicate and adoring way), can regularly yield superior outcomes over talking, over-clarifying and breaks ever will. In any case, when do you realize when you've turned out to be excessively exacting and unforgiving? Watch for these signs:

- A kid who is overly pleasant and calm since they're hesitant to commit an error.

- A youngster who is excessively delicate to even the littlest measure of analysis.

- A pitiful tyke.

- A youngster who demonstrates manifestations of moderate to severe pressure.

- A kid who is relapsing in conduct (potty preparing, freedom, problematic rest, and so forth).

In case you saw any of these signs, it might be an ideal opportunity to ease up a bit and reexamine the perfect approach to train and rebuff your youngster's lousy conduct.

Parenting Toddlers

In case you are a parent of babies, you realize how depleting life can be on an ordinary premise. There are some fundamental parenting methodologies that you can use to help influence life to be progressively reasonable when you have toddlers or youthful youngsters.

It is essential to realize how to parent your children admirably with the goal that both you and your young youngsters are more joyful and more advantageous. Rather than being overpowered by the duties and difficulties that are always being displayed, parents need to comprehend that "picking your parenting fights admirably" is generally fantastic guidance. Simplicity upon your desires and requests and figure out how to appreciate your children's extraordinary time.

Preparing

Since you realize that you need to watch out for your toddler (or the puppy may finish up with another shaded coat because of a new use of indelible marker), it very well may be hard to complete your work, for example, maintaining the house in control, cooking sound dinners. The sky is the limit from there. To keep the remainder of the house running smoothly, preparing is essential.

One approach to have solid suppers and tidbits prepared in a short time is to cut up your soil products when you return home from the market. Additionally, by making a twofold part of suppers, you can put half of the feast in the more refreshing for later use without the problem of setting it up once more.

By vacuuming, doing clothing, and other family unit errands when your toddler goes down for his rest every day, the house can likewise be kept in good condition. If you telecommute, this is also an excellent time to get up to speed with those telephone calls that require a calm family unit to finish them.

Control

Once in a while, the most challenging part about having a toddler is the consistent requirement for an order. These are the years when your sweet child figures out how to be confident out of the blue, pushing all limits with the feared word, "No!" Your toddler needs delicate, however firm, so he knows precisely where the breaking points are and that there are results each time that he/she ventures over the line. By being reliable, your toddler will discover that there is opportunity inside those limits and will step by step to quit pushing against them as regularly.

At long last, since toddlers will, in general, be debilitating, it is imperative to require investment out yourself when circumstances become difficult. It is all right to leave your screaming toddler in one room while you chill out to get it together before coming back to apply discipline.

Support self-dependence with your toddlers; however, much as could be expected. You will get a break, and they will appreciate having the option to encounter extra autonomy.

Chapter 9.

Parenting Tips for Teaching a Toddler

Toddlers can be testing and can similarly be a great deal of fun once you know how they think. Finding some crucial devices and systems to help through toddler times is all you have to appreciate this brief span. Keep in mind a little while later, and they will be on to the following stage with various difficulties for you.

There are many parenting tips for showing your toddler. The rundown is perpetual. Anyway, there are a couple of fundamental rules that can be extremely useful.

These are my five top child-rearing tips for showing your toddler. With these benchmark factors, instructing your toddler will be more straightforward.

Ensure your toddler has enough rest. We as a full capacity much better when we have had enough rest. Consider how you feel when you are overtired. It is difficult to focus; you think horrendous and attempt as you may; you can't work appropriately in some cases. Toddlers are adapting so much consistently.

Ensure you have enough rest. This is self-illustrative. You may need to reevaluate your family's rest propensities, and schedules in addition to it might take a short time to persuade it to be healthy. Anyway, the prizes will be justified, despite all the trouble. As a parent, how you feel supporting how you think and believe and, eventually, how you treat your toddler.

Have reasonable desires for both yourself and your toddler. This implies that they know about the developmental ability of your toddler. Once in a while, we can expect excessively quite a bit of them, and they aren't prepared for it yet. Now and then, we likewise expect only overly much from ourselves as parents as well. Be delicate on yourself and recall being a parent is a learning knowledge as well. This is an occupation you will learn for a mind-blowing remainder.

Take care of yourself as an individual, not just as a parent. It is anything but difficult to become involved with merely being a parent. For some, out of the blue, their toddler is the focal point of everything they do. Remember that you are an individual in your very own right. By taking care of yourself and investing significant time from your toddler consistently, you will feel invigorated. You'll even value them more. It is somewhat similar to taking an occasion from your activity. When you return, you are progressively revived, roused, and appreciate it more. Significantly, you model self-consideration to your toddler. This additionally reflects self-regard. If you don't regard yourself, you can't expect any other individual to. Be a decent good example for your little child and help them develop into self-respecting, confident grown-ups.

Be a unified front with your accomplice. If you back one another up, it shows your toddler that they can't play you off one another and undermine what every one of your states. If you don't concur at the time, bolster one another and talk about it a while later. Toddlers are brilliant and can figure out how to be manipulative in all respects right off the bat. Recall that they realize you superior to anything you do and realize how to push your catches to get what they need.

These are the pattern parenting tips for showing your toddler. When you execute different procedures for teaching your toddler to expand on these, they will be bound to be successful because these nuts and bolts are set up.

7 Tips To Unleash The Child's Creative Potential

In this section, the tips are based on the recommendations of renowned French psychologist and psychologist Michèle Freud. These tips help to unleash the creative potential of every child.

1. Support Total Freedom

Creativity is expressed when it is not repressed. Give the child complete freedom to express himself/herself. Let the child pursue interests instead of forcing him/her to sit down and finish tasks that do not cater to their needs.

One of the most critical mistakes is limiting the child's interest. Many parents mean well when they try hard to mold their child into their own concept of who he/she should be.

For example, parents often smother their child's creativity when they force them to memorize flags and country capitals. Sure, it may seem impressive for a 3-year-old to know all the flags and affluence, even all the train stops in a faraway foreign country. However, if the child isn't really interested, all that hard work will be a colossal waste. Worse, the child's potential can be seriously hampered by the adverse environment fostered by a forced activity.

Developing a child's creativity is allowing the pursuit and expression of anything that interests the child. Allow the child to use anything within his/her disposal to pursue these interests. Provide paints, brushes, easels, sports equipment, musical instruments, blocks, rings, gardening tools, etc.

Let the child pursue his/her own interests, even if it changes frequently. For example, a child may be interested in dinosaurs. Provide materials that cater to this interest. Provide toys and books. Let the child watch child-friendly shows that discuss dinosaurs. Take him/her to a trip to the museum.

If the child shifts interest to bugs, let the child pursue that as well. Do not force the child to keep working with dinosaurs. Replace available materials with ones that support this new interest.

Some parents are concerned if their child changes interests. They try to curb this by getting the child to focus only on one or two areas that they prefer. Research showed that people most likely to become Nobel Prize winners engage in multiple creative arts. Just look at Leonardo da Vinci.

He was most known as a famous painter. However, he was also an inventor. He also dabbled in medicine, with his perfect illustrations of the human body parts he observed when he dissected cadavers. Einstein is a great mathematician and scientist. He was also a fluent violinist. Einstein learned the violin then stopped for many years before taking it up again to become a fluent violinist.

2. Encourage Personal Expression

A child must have an active role in choosing what activity to pursue. Parents only work by introducing options. The child ultimately decides.

For example, parents can show the child how to play with a xylophone, drums, keyboards, guitar, and violin. Choices shouldn't stop there. They should also offer other objects such as a ball, building blocks, construction playsets, music to dance to or sing along with, paints, dolls, etc. The more choices the child has, the greater the opportunities for expression and exploration of creative potential.

Again, parents are just to help and direct the available child options. Parents should not impose what they want for their children. Creativity should be an initiative of the child.

3. Do not Judge The Quality of Results. Appreciate the Child Whatever the Results

Creativity is all about creating. It is not about reproducing what is already existing.

With these concepts in mind, parents and teachers should not judge a child's results based on others' work. The child's painting should be appreciated as it is and not compared to how another child used better colors and techniques.

Teachers and parents should also remember that a child's creative expression is precisely that—an indication of how he/she sees the world or experience the activity. It is not about having a child to play Mozart exceptionally well but more about the child expressing himself/herself through music.

What is more important is the experience and what the child learned through the experience, not an actual output to be graded, critiqued, and compared with others' work.

4. Recognize and Support Emotional Sensitivity

Children naturally fear anything new, as adults feel the same, too. Adults can help children feel more confident by explaining what to expect with an activity. Fear is significantly reduced when a person or a child knows what to expect.

With children, simple explanations may not always work. Take advantage of a child's imagination to help work out fears.

Tell a fantasy story about a hero/heroine who conquered his/her fear.

Teach the child to verbalize fear. This also helps deal with emotions. Verbalizing can start by letting the child describe what he/she feels.

Teach the child to give a name to that feeling. This way, the unseen surface starts to take on a form through that name. The child can then handle it because it has an image he/she has created for that feeling. Something known is more comfortable to hold than something faceless, nameless, and entirely unknown.

5. Support the Development of The Senses

Teaching and educating a child is more than just chanting letters and numbers, memorizing tables, and recognizing colors and shapes. Education should also be a means for a child to unleash creative potential. For this to happen, a child has to have a variety of sensory experiences.

These experiences cater to their development level. This period of discovery can be taken advantage of to help children develop and fine-tune their skills and discover and enhance their creative potential.

For example, toddlers are at a stage wherein they are just starting to discover what they can do. Learning to walk and run is an exciting time for them. Finding out that they can manipulate objects in their environment gives them a sense of awe and ride in their newly discovered capabilities.

By giving them a safe environment to move around, children become more confident to discover more about the environment and about themselves. By giving them access to objects that can help them hone their skills and express their creativity, children can find and unleash their potential.

For example, a toddler starts to learn that he/she can use his/her hands to paint with the bright, attractive paints. Give them access to toxic-free colors and provide an area where they are free to paint. This activity accomplishes two critical things. One, painting activity is fun and allows a child to practice and develop motor skills. Dipping their hands in paint and gliding them over a canvas or paper is one way to practice visual-motor skills.

The bright paints stimulate their visual sense, helping them discover the differences in colors. The paint's texture teaches them that there are different textures in the world; some are wet and cold like the paints. Some are hard like a brush. Some things are gooey. The smell can also be another sensory experience. The child becomes more exposed to different smells. This helps their brains start to distinguish the different scents.

6. Provide Freedom for Creativity

Safety is a primary consideration. However, do not overdo it. According to Michèle Freud, it is not ideal to confine children in too-safe spaces with items designed especially for them. This kind of environment produces a monotony.

Remember, again, that children are at a point in their lives where everything is new and ready to be discovered. At this stage, the child has to be exposed to various objects to discover, learn, and be creative. Monotony kills the child's initiative to discover and create. Even adults get bored with the same things every day.

Go for variety. Children at a stage where everything new and exciting. Keep feeding their excitement and give them a variety of activities and interests to pursue. Once they grasp things they can do and start to discover that they can do creativity, they will naturally come out. Soon, children will return to some of their toys and find new ways to use or play with them.

7. More on "Real" Toys Than "Educational Games"

Educational games have become a go-to for many parents. They think that these are the best toys they can give their children in order to raise them smart and creative.

According to Michèle Freud, educational toys are not exactly what parents expect them to be. In fact, these educational toys can hamper creative potential. These toys were designed to be used in specific ways only. That leaves very little room for individuality. Once the child has discovered how the education toy works, there's nothing else to do with it. There is no room for creativity. There are no opportunities to discover new ways to use the objects.

One example is a book with buttons. A child presses these buttons and sounds, such as animal sounds, are heard. These are good books for younger children because they are engaging. Parents can read books and retain the child's interest in these sounds. However, once the story has been read more than a few times, the child can get bored. The once-exciting sounds no longer hold their interest. When this time comes, the book no longer has any other use for the child. Unless, of course, years later, when the child starts to learn to read. By that time, this book may not even be appropriate for the child's age and level.

An example is a set of building blocks. It's a set that a child can see many potential ways to play with. A child can stack these largest to smallest or reverse to practice balance and size dimensions. The child can use it to build, such as a pyramid or a cube or some other project. The blocks can be used for learning geometry, for instance.

Toys like these are better than the popular educational toys in the market. These do not dictate how it can be played. Instead, it's the child who gets to think of ways, creative ways to work with them.

Chapter 10.

Consequences from Improper Training of your Toddlers

P arents must acknowledge that they are the ultimate reference materials for their children. To this end, the parenting method adopted in the children's training has long-term and short-term effects on them. In this chapter, you'll be shown some of the general consequences that follow your toddlers' improper parenting. According to the 2011 report by the UK's Department of Education, it is understood that the conduct of children who had improper parental guidance been twice as worse as the average child. This was traced to inappropriate parenting involving physical punishment, verbal abuse, coercion, lack of interaction, and inadequate supervision.

Greater Vulnerability to Psychological Disorders

In a child development journal, it is understood that children who are directly or indirectly exposed to physical or verbal abuse at their early age have a higher risk of having psychological disorders. In this study, there was no prevalence when psychological diseases are placed in comparison. However, these psychological disorders were all traced to factors in the early stage of children's development. It was found that the relationships with siblings in the family they come from, or relationships with their parents had been damaged. According to the Child Abuse & Neglect Journal, studies show that children who have been victims of abuse display post-traumatic stress disorder for a substantial period of their lifetime.

Defiance to Laws

Because of a research article published in the International Journal of Child, Youth and Family Studies, it is found that children who suffered parental negligence in their early days were more susceptible to being charged for juvenile delinquency. In this study, researchers were directed to investigate the connection between parental oversight and juvenile delinquency. Although, some of the intellectual gaps identified in that study have been filled in other studies.

One of these studies is the research published in Behavioral Sciences & the Law Journal. In that study, it was found that mothers who had once been charged with juvenile delinquency commonly give birth to or nurture children with antisocial attitudes and tendencies to defy laws. According to the study, this was traced to parental abuse and negligence. In such cases, the problems of defiance to laws may be generational.

Depression

In the 'Annual Reviews' the publication titled, "Parenting and Its Effects on Children: On Reading and Misreading Behavior Genetics," Professor Eleanor E. Maccoby of Stanford University explains that one of the causal factors of depression in children is parental adverse reactions towards their children. This line of thinking was also contained in a National Institute of Health journal submission by Danielle In the article, H. Dallaire, "Relation of Positive and Negative Parenting to Children's Depressive Symptoms." With these distinctive, credible reports reaching similar conclusions, it is hard to doubt that it is indeed proper that factors such as overall support, verbal condemnation, physical punishment, and even depression of the parents are causal to the depression of a child.

Failure to Thrive

One of the implications of failure to thrive in toddlers is the retardation of mental growth, physical growth, and the possibility of malnutrition. According to research submitted to the American Journal of Orthopsychiatry, it was learned that failure to thrive in toddlers is ultimately linked to parental negligence. Children who are victims of "failure to thrive" are found to have lacked good nutrition that is essential for healthy growth. This reduces their standard growth rate. A publication in the journal Pediatrics also traced the failure to thrive syndrome in toddlers to medical child abuse. It is found that parents who impose unnecessary medical treatments on their children make them vulnerable to the syndrome. In cases where your toddlers find it difficult to thrive, you need to check the medical procedures you have been exposing them to and the measure of care you show them.

Aggression

According to Rick Nauert's Psych Central article, "Negative Parenting Style Contributes to Child Aggression," the various research conducted by different specialists at the University of Minnesota all had similar conclusions; toddlers who were aggressive and quick to anger all had poor interactions with their mothers. The conclusion was that one of the effects of bad parenting on toddlers is an aggression on the children's part. The mothers studied treated their children aggressively, were verbally hurtful, and harmful towards their children. The more negative parenting, the greater the child's aggression to colleagues. This created a certain level of hostility between mothers and toddlers. Though, more research is now invested into knowing whether the relationship of the toddlers' fathers with their mothers influence on the bad conduct of the mothers towards their children is.

Poor Academic Performance

One of the consequences of parental neglect is the gross reduction in the toddlers' academic performance. This view is credited to a study conducted and published in the Child Abuse and Neglect Journal.

The study concludes that when parents have minimal interactions with their children, it impairs the children's' learning ability compared to their peers. The children also lack social relationships. Further research shows that neglect is no less disastrous than physical abuse in terms of the toddlers' academic performance.

According to another study in the journal Demography, children whose parents frequently relocate or migrate also tend to poor performance in school. The truth is constant relocation is usually a factor that is above the power of the parents. Nonetheless, it may have detrimental consequences on the child's educational growth.

In terms of children's mathematical performance, research has shown that the parents' mathematical interests can determine whether they are good at it. According to Melissa E. Libertus, an Associate Professor at the University of Pittsburgh said the connection is either environmental or hereditary. In this light, parents that are easily provoked at their child's academic performance in mathematics should know it might have genetic or ecological causes. Having seen some of the behavioral, cognitive and social consequences of improper parenting, it is time you were introduced to a grand principle for training your toddlers.

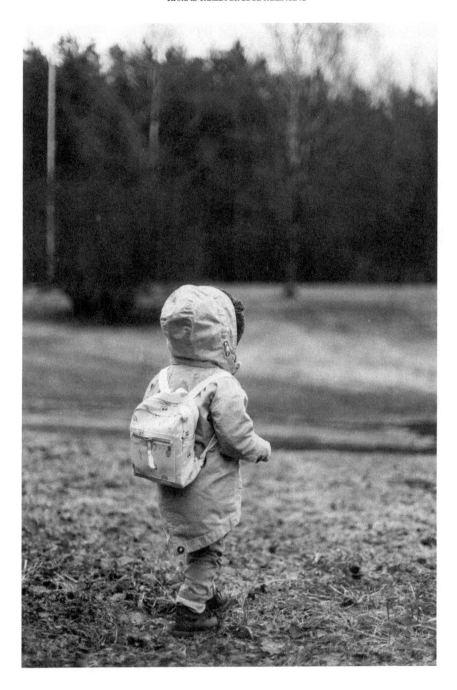

Chapter 11.

Montesssori Method Managing Choice and

Freedom

I n my experience as a teacher, I found that many students came into the classroom, knowing exactly what they wanted to work on. If there was a science experiment going on in the corner, many students would come in and check on that first. Others would head straight to the reading corner. Some students loved to see what the latest materials were on the practical life shelves in the preschool classroom. Nearly all of them loved beginning sewing lessons. Throughout the day, children move from one activity to the next in a series of decisions they make largely on their own. Students are invited to presentations with the teacher who carefully guides and orchestrates the activity in the classroom.

Choice and freedom in the classroom can be overwhelming for some students, hindering their productivity and ability to progress. This can happen for both neurotypical and children with ASD. What can we do to support choice and freedom at home and at school?

In this chapter, we'll discuss the importance of freedom and choice in Montessori and learn why this can be challenging for ASD students.

Then, I'll offer some strategies for increasing your child's ability to manage freedom and choice.

Freedom and Choice in the Montessori Method

In our lives as adults, we make decisions frequently. It's an essential survival skill. But, even many adults struggle with choices. For example, prioritizing a task list incorrectly can mean you need to stay up late to finish a project due at work the next day. Or, a struggle to choose what to purchase at the grocery store can reveal that we haven't prepared ahead of time with a meal plan or even taken a quick inventory of the pantry. These seemingly mundane skills all boil down to choices we make that can enhance or add stress to our lives.

The Montessori method aims to prepare students to handle complex decision-making from the very beginning of their schooling. Beginning with choice in activities (as long as certain routines and rules such as cleaning up are being followed), students are slowly given more responsibility. In the elementary years, Montessori students are encouraged to organize and execute field trips to nearby attractions or community institutions. By middle school, they might plan a trip that lasts a few days and involves several travel hours. The ultimate goal? Confident adults who are skilled at managing decisions in their lives, from buying groceries to making career choices.

How does freedom manifest itself exactly? Every Montessori classroom is unique. Yet, they all have the thread of freedom in common that's a function of the classroom setup and teachers' guidance. Shelves of materials, books, and command cards are arranged according to the subject area. After receiving a presentation, children are free to work with the material as they please, as long as another child isn't using it. Starting in elementary grades, lists, work plans, or student-teacher meetings are sometimes used to help track progress.

This ability to handle freedom responsibly doesn't come automatically. Rules and routines are taught in the classroom so that students know the classroom expectations. Using a rug or table for work, cleaning up each material after using it, and placing it correctly when done is basic. Students must also use a quiet voice in the classroom, avoid disturbing others, and wait their turn to use materials that others are using. Only some materials and activities can be used or done in pairs or groups.

The Prepared Environment

Why did Montessori include this element in her classroom design? In addition to believing that freedom and choice are important life skills to learn how to handle, she also knew that allowing space in the classroom also goes hand in hand with following the child. You can't follow the child if they are entirely restricted. Montessori carefully orchestrated the freedom and choices that children would have in the classroom.

She did this by building a prepared environment, the classroom, for the children she was working with. Distractions were kept to a minimum, with no loud, glitzy posters or excessive noise. Instead, the children's attention was drawn towards the learning materials, which were the most exciting.

Create Structure With a Chart

When a child arrives as a newcomer to a Montessori program, it's not uncommon to limit choices. Having the child use items from an individual shelf or providing additional guidance and support when picking materials is quite familiar. For children with ASD, this approach is a good start, but working out a routine and representing that visually is often the most helpful. For pre-literate or non-verbal children, images, or pictures of the materials used can be printed to create the schedule. These sorts of supports can be beneficial for adapting to this new way of doing things.

Also, some children may benefit from additional structure. For example, Lois Ormonde noted that she and her student often used a silent timer to encourage him to complete tasks. I also noticed the difference between two students on the ASD spectrum during my time teaching in the lower elementary classroom. While one student struggled to finish tasks, another finished them without any external intervention at all. However, the first student was highly motivated by creating a checklist of the work he wanted to complete and then crossing off each activity as he finished it.

Likely, be a different, unique solution for each child with autism. All children are individual, and what motivates them, makes them tick, and makes learning enjoyable.

Slowly Offer Choice

Over time, you can gradually offer the child some choice in the activities. First, you might provide that the child changes the order of the routine. Or, you may consider offering two new materials and have the child choose which one to try that day. In this way, the child slowly takes more control over their learning.

Why offer the choice if things are going well with structure and support? The externally imposed system requires constant reliance on an adult or outside force to regulate what's going on. To achieve true independence, children must be able to make decisions and make use of freedoms. By starting in a safe, controlled environment and slowly shifting the responsibility of choices to the child, greater independence is achieved.

Observe

Make sure you keep observing the child, ensure that needs are being met. For example, you may discover that a weekly schedule should also be posted somewhere in the room for the child to see in addition to a daily schedule. Or, perhaps you'll learn that the child is very motivated in some academic areas and can be allowed more excellent choice within specific subject areas. Most importantly, the child should be viewed as the leading indicator of what's working well or not so well. Changing several items in a routine at once could be stressful for one child, but could mean improvements for another. With careful observation, you can help guide a shift to greater independence and freedom.

Allow Observing

A critical element of a Montessori classroom is the opportunity that the children have to observe one another. Children are free to watch another child working, as long as they are respectful and don't interfere. Montessori believed that this was a vital motivating factor, especially for the younger students in the mixed-age classroom. Many students with autism, as well as neurotypical children, benefit greatly from observing. In addition to Montessori's insights on keeping in the school, a wealth of autism experts and organizations agree that allowing students to watch before being asked to try something can be very helpful. Lois Ormonde shared, "What worked for my student was I would model what he should do. Then, he would practice until he could do it." The organization, Montessori Education for Autism, also agrees, arguing that some students with autism may engage in "third party participation," observing other students use a material many times. Even if the child never decides to use the material on their own, they can benefit from this interaction.

While limits on observing should be imposed when children interrupt or distract others. Children with autism can become unobtrusive observers and gain much from the ability to stand-by and watch others when participating is too tricky. Over time, with guidance, most children can gain greater independence and make more and more choices in the classroom or their education. By empowering children to make decisions with regards to their knowledge, their agency can be increased.

CPSIA information can be obtained
at www.ICGtesting.com
Printed in the USA
BVHW062004250321
603411BV00002B/130

9 781914 421396